C000136244

OpenAdoption
OpenMind

BOOK THREE of the
GLASS HALF-FULL PARENTING PERPECTIVES series

BOOK THREE of the
GLASS HALF-FULL PARENTING PERSPECTIVES series

Open Adoption
Open Mind

an adoptive father's
inspiring true story

RUSSELL ELKINS

Open Adoption, Open Mind: An Adoptive Father's Inspiring True Story
Book three in the Glass Half-Full Adoption Memoirs series
By Russell Elkins
©2019 Russell Elkins

Some of the names in this book have been changed to protect the privacy of the individuals involved.

Chief line editor: Jenna Lovell
Content editing team: Jenna Lovell, Kim Foster, Martin Casey, Cathy Watson Childs

Cover photo and author photo by Jammie Elkins Photography
Cover design by Inky's Nest Design
Interior book design by Inky's Nest Design

ISBN: 978-0-9899873-9-4

Inky's Nest Publishing

RussellElkins.com
1st edition
First printed in 2019 in the United States of America

CONTENTS

To all the wonderful birthparents out there.
I hope the whole world sees and learns from your strength.

1

HIDING WITH THE GOLDFISH

We had only come to the pet store to find a new goldfish, but we found ourselves in quite the predicament when I happened to turn around in time to see Darcie and her husband cross the aisle ten feet in front of me. I froze. This was the last thing we wanted to happen.

Our daughter, Hazel, was five years old at that time and it had been three years since we had last been in contact with her birthmother, Darcie. The last form of communication between us was in the form of a letter she had hand-delivered in the night to our home and left on our doorstep for us to find in the morning. She had not minced words in what she wrote. Although she had previously felt comfortable enough to stop by our home two or three times a week, she made it perfectly clear in her letter that she had no interest in ever seeing or talking to us again.

So there we were, cornered in the back area of the pet store by the fish tanks. There was only one way out of there, which would cause us to have to walk right past Darcie and her husband. Our expectation was that they would quickly find what they were looking for and be out of the store within a few minutes, but that turned out not to be the case. They were obviously in no hurry.

We spent half an hour looking at all the different types of fish and trying to keep our voices down. Half an hour! Young kids can only stare at fish for so long before they begin to get restless, and the inevitable happened.

"Daddy, I have to go to the bathroom," Hazel said.

"You can't hold it?"

"No. I need to go to the bathroom."

We were not scared of Darcie or her husband. We also were not afraid of getting ourselves into an uncomfortable situation. After all, what could be more uncomfortable than hunkering down in the back of a pet store for half an hour hoping we would not be seen?

Our reason for trying to avoid them was because of how we respected and loved them just as much as we always had. As I said before, Darcie had made it perfectly clear that she was not interested in ever seeing us again and we knew that this chance encounter would be uncomfortable for her. We did not want to put her through that if we could avoid it.

I scooped Hazel into my arms, took a deep breath, and started our way toward the bathroom. Any hope of passing them without being recognized was soon gone. I kept my eyes down on the floor as I walked briskly past. I heard Darcie's voice talking playfully with her husband as we passed their aisle, but in my mind's eye I could picture her facial expression when I heard her voice cut off in mid-sentence.

Jammie and our son, Ira, were waiting for us just outside the bathroom a few minutes later.

"Are they gone now?" I asked.

"Darcie hurried out the door as soon as she saw you. Her husband is at the checkout stand right now paying for things," Jammie said.

That moment was really uncomfortable for us, but that day turned out to be another turning point in our adoption story with Darcie. But before I tell how that day changed our path, I should probably rewind back to where *Open Adoption, Open Arms* (book two in this series) left off and recount how we got to this point in the first place.

When that book left off, Darcie had taken a few months off from seeing us to try to get her social life back on track. When she began visiting again, we did not know how often to expect her visits. The location of her new job caused her to drive within a mile of our house multiple times each day. That meant she would have to make the same decision multiple times a day about whether or not to drop in to see us. We had grown so comfortable together that she was granted permission to drop by whenever she pleased, like any other friend. She was coming by two or three times a week at that point—sometimes on her lunch break and other times after work.

There was an innate problem with that. Open adoption relationships, even when they are going well, carry with them an increased intensity. That intensity between us was a good intensity, but it was an intensity nonetheless. When someone stops by for a visit, we would inevitably drop whatever we were doing to give that person our undivided attention. Having that open invitation to stop by without advanced notice created a situation where we were always wondering if she would stop by. Although we loved her deeply, wondering all day every day if she was going to stop by continuously put us on edge. That was not a fun way to live.

When Hazel was a little over a year old, we were invited to a large gathering for Darcie's family. About thirty of Darcie's aunts, uncles, siblings, and cousins showed up to her house for a barbecue. Jammie and I decided we would pull Darcie aside at the end of the evening to discuss our need for a few boundaries regarding visits to our home.

We explained to her our reasons and she said she understood. We gave her the power to decide how often she would like to visit and for how long, but we just wanted those visits to be planned out in advance.

Darcie decided to mull over that decision for a few days before settling on a schedule. A few days later, when she came to our house on another lunchtime visit, she informed us that she had been looking back on how things had progressed in her life regarding the adoption and her personal life and she could see that everything was still revolving closely around Hazel and our adoption situation. She knew she needed to take another break. This time, instead of continuing to receive pictures and updates during her break like she had done before, she wanted to take a break from everything—pictures, updates, visits... everything. Just for a little while. Just so she could break herself from the need to have her life so intertwined with ours.

That was not exactly what we had been going for, but if that was what she needed, then we were happy to honor her wish.

She said she would probably take about three months off, but three months came and went without having contact. When we reached out, she informed us that the time away had been good for her and that she was not quite ready yet to start visiting or receiving regular updates.

It was during that time that she met the man who would become her husband. After about six months of having almost no contact, she sent us a text message saying she would like to see us again and asked if we would like to go out to dinner with her and her boyfriend. We began visiting again, but visits were not nearly as frequent or unpredictable as before. It was nice.

Darcie and her husband chose to have a small wedding ceremony with only close friends and family in attendance. Jammie and I felt honored to be part of that day as we celebrated this big milestone. As we expected to happen, this new chapter in her life also meant that she would pull away a little more.

Open adoption can be really hard at times. As Westley in *The Princess Bride* said, "Anyone who says otherwise is selling something." That first year was definitely the most difficult, but that did not mean that things got easy after that year had gone by.

Somewhere around the time of Hazel's second birthday things were going well with Darcie, but then something happened to cause a rift between us. It must have been something relatively minor because I do not even remember what it was. The real issue was not whatever it was that happened between us that day, but the real issue turned out to be the way we all handled it.

Jammie and I were very busy in the adoption advocacy community at that time. We were running a web page where anybody could come to discuss various aspects of adoption. More than a thousand people would visit our page each day from countries all around the world to take part in a discussion, seek advice and find comradery. We were aware of other similar forums that would only discuss the beautiful sides of open adoption, and some others that only centered on the hot and controversial topics. Jammie and I tried our best to focus on what we considered to be real. We did not want people to believe open adoption was always roses and hugs, and we did not want people to associate adoption only with controversy either. We tried to present a healthy balance of topics where people could discuss the difficult sides of adoption while still seeing its overall beauty.

We posted something about our current struggle on the page with hopes of sparking some good conversation as well as get some quality feedback. That was our biggest mistake. Darcie felt like we were airing our dirty laundry out to the world, and in hindsight it is not hard to see why she viewed it that way. Typing our disagreement onto our page where the world could see it poured gasoline onto the fire. Over the next two days, anything we said only fanned the flames. That was what drove her to write that angry letter—the one that made it perfectly clear that she never wanted to see or speak to us again.

We immediately wished we could somehow take it back, but the damage was done.

Jammie and I were devastated. Her letter pierced us right through the heart because of how much we loved Darcie. We did not want her out of our life and we did not want her out of Hazel's life. We were heartbroken that she not only pulled away, but that she did it so angrily. This was a very different feeling than when she was taking time away to rebuild her personal and social life.

As time went by, I came to wonder if this outcome was inevitable. Jammie and I were not perfect. We never claimed to be. With our relationship being so intensely and intimately intertwined the way it was for those first two years, we were bound to make a mistake. If we had not messed things up that day or in that way, it would have probably been only a matter of time before we slipped in some other way. Through the gift of hindsight, I could see how delicate our situation always was.

Three years went by and we found ourselves cornered in that pet store by the fish tanks hoping to avoid an uncomfortable confrontation. When Jammie and I got back to our car, we sat for a few minutes in the parking lot reminiscing on how much we missed Darcie and wished things could have gone differently between us.

Although we never spoke or made eye contact in that pet store, the incident must have churned her emotions because we received an email from Darcie just a few days later. This was the first time she had reached out to us in any way since leaving that letter on our doorstep. She expressed a desire to see Hazel again, but we could easily tell she had not completely forgiven us for how we had wronged her years earlier. As much as we wanted Hazel to have a personal relationship with her birthmother again, our family is a package deal. The idea of Darcie bonding with our daughter while resenting Jammie and me simply did not work.

In our reply, we conveyed our need to work things out between us adults first. If Darcie was interested, our preference was to begin again by spending a little time together without the children present—perhaps meeting somewhere for dinner—and then later down the road we could discuss face-to-face visits with Hazel again when the time was right.

Our desire to hold off on visiting with Hazel was not solely based on our need for Darcie to let go of her resentment toward us. I will get into this subject more in the next chapter, but Hazel has always been both highly sentimental and very pensive, even at five years old. Hazel missed Darcie. Although her memories of her were extremely limited, she talked about Darcie often. We know our daughter well enough to know that, as much as she missed her birthmom, it would have been much worse to have Darcie come back into her life only to leave again. She would have been devastated.

Darcie did not accept our dinner invitation at that time, but said she needed to consider it.

A few months later, my band performed a two hour set at the county fair in the same small town where Hazel had been born. After the show, we bought a bunch of overpriced carnival ride tickets for Hazel and Ira to squander. As we stood in line for a kiddie-sized roller coaster, I heard Jammie talking to someone behind me.

"Oh my goodness. Can I give you a hug?" Jammie said.

I turned around to see a petite lady looking at Jammie with a confused expression on her face. "Why?" the lady asked.

"Because my daughter is your granddaughter," Jammie said. "It's us. Jammie and Russell."

Her mouth dropped open as recognition set in. "Oh my," she said, and she held out her arms.

We talked for a few minutes before sharing another hug and wishing each other well. I felt bad that Hazel seemed much more interested in the roller coaster she was about to ride than she was in her biological grandma whom she had not seen since before she had learned to walk, but it was a nice encounter.

We kept our eye on Grandma and made sure to approach her for one last hug before we left the fair. This time Hazel was not so fixated on the carnival ride, and by this time Grandma had joined up with Darcie's sister as well.

A few days after that chance encounter, we received another email from Darcie. This time she focused more on catching up on our lives than anything else. She and her husband had a son now. She had finished her nursing degree and was now a full-time RN. She talked about the sweet as well as the sour that had gone on in their life over the past few years. In the end, she said she was not quite ready for visits again (not with Hazel or with us alone), but she just wanted to reconnect through email.

We sent a reply along with some current pictures of our family. Contact has slowly grown more frequent with time. After spending those uncomfortable years apart, we have had to rebuild our relationship anew from the ground up, but that is what we are doing. The days of feeling it would be best to avoid contact by hiding by the goldfish are gone.

During the earlier days after Hazel's adoption, updates had been pretty one-sided with us sharing with Darcie the things going on in our life. Things are different now because updates go both ways. She sends us pictures and updates of her beautiful family as well (she and her husband now have two children).

We still have not met face-to-face since those early days, but recent emails have caused me to believe she has forgiven us for our mistake. The most recent email we received was especially beautiful, expressing how she has come to realize how much she misses us—all of us, not just Hazel. The feeling is mutual. We love her. I do not know when, but I believe the day will come when we are all ready to visit again. We look forward to that day, but we do not want to rush something that important.

2

OUR ROCK

Hazel's birthfather, Caleb, has been a rock for us since day one. He has been the epitome of what open adoption should be. And by that, I mean that he has been open to the need for change even when we were sure he wished things could remain the same.

During the first few years, Caleb would make the five-hour drive to come spend the afternoon together before driving back in the evening. He did that a couple of times a year in the beginning. His parents even made the drive to visit us a few times without him. Any time we knew we were going to be in eastern Idaho, we would contact them beforehand and we would get together with him and his extended family.

When Hazel was little, the amount of contact between families was completely dependent upon whatever Jammie and I organized with Caleb. We knew that the day would come when we would need to start tailoring those visits according to her needs, not ours. We did not know at what age that would happen. When it did happen, we did not know if she would express a desire for more contact or less.

The time to make a change manifested itself during the summer after Hazel turned four years old. It happened when we visited with Caleb and his family three times within a five week period.

Those three visits kicked off with Caleb's parents coming to town. His mother is an elementary school teacher and she was required to come to Boise for a training course. They spent the evening with us in our home before leaving to sleep at a hotel.

Months before that visit, we had already planned to make a trip to visit them in eastern Idaho. We expected this visit to be a bigger event than we typically had with them. We invited aunts and uncles and cousins and all sorts of good people. Caleb's parents offered us the guest room in their home to spend the night, which we happily accepted. The evening was full of horseback riding, barbecuing and playing guitar out back by the fire pit.

A few weeks after that visit to eastern Idaho, Caleb's job required he come here to Boise for two days. He spent a little time doing things for his work and a lot of time with us. We filled the day with a fun trip to the zoo. That night we brought out the popcorn and enjoyed a movie. Caleb spent the night on an air mattress in our living room. We cooked a nice breakfast and spent the morning together before he headed back home around lunchtime.

The aftermath of that last visit was quite different than any we'd had with him in all of the previous years.

First of all, when talking solely about how Jammie and I were feeling, it drained us. It had been a few years since Darcie had last visited and Brianna lived so far away that we were not able to see her very often. We had grown accustomed to feeling a bit of distance from our adoptions. Even though we had visited together quite a few times with Caleb, the nature of our relationship still carried an innate feeling of needing to prove Caleb had made the right choice when he decided to place Hazel into our home. As we always did when we were going to have a special guest spend the night in our home, we scrubbed the house from top to bottom. Although he was not asking for much with his visit, we still felt responsible for his well-being, which led to us paying an unreasonable amount of attention to how we thought he was feeling at every moment. Spending so much time together over a five week period brought back old feelings of exhaustion we had not felt around adoption since the kids were younger.

Although we felt fatigued from the intense nature of the relationship, the greater issues that surfaced were those surrounding Hazel. She was only four-years-old, which meant she was old enough to realize there was a difference in who Caleb was—someone different than any other person in her life. Her uncles all adored her, but they did not dote on her quite like this. When she was near him, she was not just a little girl, she was a princess.

It was not hard to see it begin to go to her head. Not only did she pick up on the fact that Caleb treated her differently than any other man in her life, but she also perceived that Jammie and I treated her differently while he was near. Few things are as uncomfortable for parents as having to deal with an all-out tantrum in the presence of birthparents. Especially while Caleb was still in our home, as all young children would do, she began to push the boundaries as far as she could to see what she could get away with. But it did not stop after he went back home to eastern Idaho. She was insufferable for at least two weeks after those three visits. That was not her nature. She had always been such a sweet-hearted little girl.

On top of how the environmental contrast pushed her to behave differently than she typically did at home, I found myself battling different emotions than I was accustomed to feeling regarding Caleb. There was nothing wrong with him treating her like a princess. That was expected. It was hard for me to watch Hazel prefer that over the relationship she and I had. She had always been a very affectionate little girl. When she let go of my hand at the zoo to run up to Caleb and slip her hand into his, I felt a jolt of jealousy that I had never felt around him before. If that were to have happened only once or twice during the visits, I doubt it would have affected me very much, but it happened often during every activity as well as during down time. In the back of my mind, she was supposed to always prefer my hand over anyone else's (except Jammie's, of course).

I loved Caleb. I did not enjoy feeling this way around him. Those contrasting feelings beat me up as his presence pulled me in two different directions. Those feelings had not surfaced like this when she was younger. This was new to me.

As difficult as those aspects were, however, the greatest concern for us manifested over the following weeks. As I mentioned earlier, Hazel was a pensive little girl—especially for a four-year-old. She would periodically come to Jammie or me with the types of questions a young girl could not possibly understand.

"Who is Jocelyn's birthdad?" she asked one day.

"Jocelyn doesn't have a birthdad like you do," Jammie said. "Jocelyn's dad is Uncle Clark."

"I know her dad is Uncle Clark, but who is her birthdad?"

"Not everybody has a dad and a birthdad like you do. Most people don't."

Explaining the concept of birthfather proved to be more difficult than we had anticipated. We had been able to explain adoption and birthmothers by telling her that she had grown in Darcie's tummy but that Darcie was not ready to be a mother at that time. We told her we were not able to grow a baby in Jammie's tummy because "Mommy's tummy is broken," but we wanted to raise kids more than anything in this world. This simple explanation brought adoption and birthmothers down to her level and she was able to accept it in her own way, but it still did not explain Caleb.

It seemed the more we tried to explain Caleb without getting into the birds and the bees with a four-year-old, the more we confused her. But most of her questions were not in regards to the "hows" of a birthfather, but focused more on the "whys." Why was she so special to him? He did not live nearby like Uncle Clark did. Why did he did not have any other kids if he loves kids like he does her?

Hazel has a tendency to laser focus her mind on concepts she cannot understand or which unsettle her. The concept of birthfather did both of these things.

For example, a while later, after she began attending public kindergarten, she came home from school with a solemn look on her face. Her personality is typically very bubbly, so it was not hard to notice something was weighing on her as she sat quietly during dinner.

"Mom, Dad, is Santa Claus real?" she asked.

In our home, we like the fun of having Santa Claus be part of our Christmas. We wanted to keep that tradition for at least a couple more years.

"What do you think, Hazel?" Jammie said. "Do you think he is real?"

She pondered for a moment. "Yes."

"Then that's what matters," Jammie said.

"But Gracie says he isn't real," Hazel said.

"It's okay if Gracie doesn't believe Santa Claus is real," Jammie said. "She's allowed to believe that. But we get to believe what we choose to believe, and so in our home Santa Claus is real."

I am sure that type of conversation happens every December in homes all across the globe, but Hazel could not leave it there. The next day she came home from school with the same question, which sparked the same conversation. And the next day. And the next day. Each day the weight on her shoulders seemed heavier than the day before.

We finally decided we had better bring both kids in the living room for a talk. We brought Ira in on the conversation too because we felt it would have been weird telling Hazel that Santa Claus was not real while her older brother still did not know.

"Kids, do you believe Santa Claus is real?" I asked.

Hazel shrugged her shoulders.

Ira said "yes" in such a way that made it clear he was thinking, "Of course he is. Duh. What kind of stupid question is that?"

"Well, we can see how the idea of Santa Claus has been stressing Hazel out lately, so we decided now was the time to tell you the truth about him."

Hazel's eyes grew wider while Ira looked at us with that facial expression of complete confusion.

"Santa Claus is a tradition around Christmastime that is supposed to be a fun tradition, but we can see that it is stressing you out too much, which kind of sucks all the fun out of it." And we went on to explain the truth about Santa Claus.

This experience with Santa Claus was similar to trying to explain Caleb, except that there was no way of finally breaking the news and telling her the truth once we decided she had stressed over it enough. We tried coming at it from a slightly different angle every time she brought it up, but each conversation brought the same result: confusion. A lot of the time she would simply walk away in the middle of the conversation, sometimes while we were still in mid-sentence. I distinctly remember one day when she cupped both hands over her ears and said, "My ears hurt," before turning to walk away.

Having had her in the presence of Caleb and his family so much over a five week span meant that her questions and emotions had not been given sufficient time to simmer back to normal before being around them again.

The fact that Ira's birthmother was still a part of our lives but Darcie was nowhere to be found only boggled her mind more.

It was clear to us that we had pushed her four-year-old brain too far that summer. Open adoption can be very difficult in that aspect. We have to figure things out as we go along. Each relationship with birthparents and their families is different. Ira and Hazel both conceptualize and react to the idea of adoption very differently. Ira did not stress about adoption or birthparents in the same way Hazel did, not even when Brianna came to stay with us for a weeklong visit. All we could do was try our best to do what we felt was right for our children and for our family, and then make adjustments as we went.

One difficult part about this situation was that we had grown quite comfortable around Caleb and his family. They have always been wonderful to us. Having such an open relationship with them made it difficult for us to come out say we needed to pull away from them for a little while. To Caleb, this had to feel like he had been blindsided. That was never our intention, and although we made an attempt to explain our reasons, I doubt he fully understood. How could he understand without being there to watch her turmoil over those weeks following his visits? Still, he honored our wish.

After making that request, we could sense his hesitancy over the next few years. He has always been the kind of man who would not want to step on our toes or ask for something that would make us uncomfortable. Consequently, the fact that we told him we had to take a step back meant that it was hard for him to know where things stood at all times. Any time he asked for anything, he worried whether or not he was asking too much.

We still visited together. We still made the five hour drive out to see him and welcomed his large family to the event, but we did not stay overnight with them and we did not do it quite as often.

Caleb has progressed a lot with his life over the last few years. We are very proud to call him part of our family. He graduated from college and has a great career going for him. We were elated when we found out that he proposed to his girlfriend. We had been able to meet her on a few occasions and they are perfect together.

When we pulled back on visits, we knew it would be temporary. Now that Hazel is a little older, she is processing things better than when she was four. We expect to see Caleb a little more this coming summer than we have over the last few years. In our church, children are considered old enough to choose baptism once they reach eight-years-old, so we have already invited Caleb and his extended family to the event. Caleb has also invited us to come his way to be part of his wedding.

Our goal has always been to attempt to be as consistent as possible. Unfortunately, as has been the case with Caleb, consistency is sometimes too much to ask for in an open adoption relationship. We had found ourselves wanting to be more and more open with time, but there came that summer when we realized we had pushed that relationship a bit too far and had to backtrack for Hazel's sake as well as our own.

Right now things are as healthy and well-balanced as ever. As bouncy as the ride has been, the one consistency in the whole ordeal has been Caleb. He has been our rock, and we are eternally grateful that he has the ability to always be that for our Hazel May.

3

AN EVERCHANGING AND UNHEALTHY RELATIOSHIP

When the second book of this series wrapped up, we still had not been in direct contact with Daren. The last time he was part of our story was when he surprised Ira's birthmother with court papers. Those legal issues fell flat almost as soon as they began, but that part of our story sure shook us up. And to top it off, the last we had heard anything from him was because he was still going out of his way to harass Brianna.

Our plan was never to keep him out of our family. We reached out to him a handful of times but eventually gave up. That all changed when Ira was about four-years-old.

Daren's mother emailed us and asked for some pictures. She also asked if she could be one of our "friends" on Facebook. Our preference since the early days of our adoption story had been for contact to be centered around our children's biological parents and nobody else—not around any of their friends

29

or even their close family. So, the fact that this was Daren's mother contacting us and not Daren forced us to make a decision: We would need to turn her away and say that Daren would be the one who needed to ask for updates, or we could break from the way we had always done things. Our reasons for doing so were laid out in greater detail in the first book of this series, but suffice it to say that open adoption is complicated enough as it is. Steering around the birthparents to communicate with other people only served to complicate the situation even further.

We decided to break from our norm. Jammie accepted her Facebook friend request and sent Daren's mother some pictures and updates. Receiving those pictures must have overloaded her emotions because things exploded immediately afterward. I cannot understand why she would think this type of behavior would be tolerable, but she immediately began writing nasty messages about Brianna all over her Facebook page. That was unacceptable. Nobody talks about our Brianna that way.

So that was it. We told her we had already broken from our norm when we decided to bring her into our circle without Daren wanting to be part of it as well, and the only thing she did was prove why we had made that decision in the first place.

We had no more contact with Daren or his family for about another year before something very unexpected happened: Daren began to show interest in Ira and in our family. Even more unexpected than that was that he contacted Brianna with an apology. I had always figured he would want to have some sort of contact with us someday, but I never expected him to apologize to Brianna for how things had gone in their past.

Brianna wrote to us and informed us that he had asked for our phone numbers so he could send us a text message. We were taken aback, but the fact that he was showing signs of maturity as well as a greater ability to be respectful piqued our curiosity, if nothing else. Our response was to ask Brianna how she felt about it, to which she responded with an open mind.

Over the next few weeks, we shared a little about ourselves, including pictures of Ira and our family. Within a few weeks of that contact, we reached out to Daren's mother and offered her pictures as well. Now that the door was open between us and Daren, we felt a little more comfortable with the idea of having other relatives in on the mix. Of course, we also made it crystal clear that Brianna was our girl through and through, and we would not tolerate the type of disrespect we had seen last time we were in contact. She agreed.

Daren was in his early twenties now and no longer lived at home with his parents. He had just become father to a baby girl. I think the shock of having a new baby in his arms jolted his mind into thinking about Ira in different ways than he had in the past.

That line of communication with Daren stayed the same for a few years. We randomly exchanged text messages. We sent pictures via email. We uploaded pictures and updates to a blog for him to download and print. We connected with him as well as a few of his close family on Facebook.

I could never say we got to the point of having a fully open or close relationship with Daren like we have enjoyed with Brianna, Caleb or Darcie, but it was nice while it lasted.

Everything came crashing down one morning.

It began with Jammie sending Daren a text message to wish him a happy birthday (text messages were his preferred form of communication). His first response was confusing, followed by another one that sent our minds spinning. He began asking Jammie inappropriate questions about herself.

"It kind of sounds like he doesn't realize who he's chatting with," I said as I stared at her phone.

"Do you think that's it?" she asked.

I shrugged. "Probably. You didn't sign your name on any of the texts. I think he thinks you're someone else."

Jammie texted Daren again to ask if he realized who she was. He responded, "Of course I do," and proceeded to ask another question that was even more inappropriate than the previous one.

She texted back again, this time asking if he was high.

He said he was not, and before too long he asked if she would be willing to send an inappropriate photo of herself. We could not believe what we were reading.

"I still don't think he knows who he is talking with," I said. "Nobody is that stupid."

So Jammie texted again. He beat around the bush a couple of times before Jammie insisted. "Prove to me you know who I am. How do we know each other?" Jammie texted.

"You're Ira's mom," Daren texted back.

That was all we needed to know. Any respect we had for him was gone. And just as bad, we could not help but feel like any respect he had ever claimed to have for us was only an act.

I know I should have probably been crazy mad at Daren that day, but all of those feelings were overshadowed by pity. How sad that a man's mind could be that distorted that he would risk throwing away an important relationship for something like that.

We closed that door for a while, but have since allowed it to be cracked open again. We have sent a few updates and pictures since then, but we are not connected on Facebook anymore. We also have sent his mother a few small things here and there, but contact is not frequent or extensive with any of them.

I suppose anything is possible in the future, but I do not expect to ever have a close relationship with Daren, and I do not expect him to be much of a positive influence in Ira's life.

4

~

SO GROWN UP

In just a few months it will have been ten years since Brianna first contacted us. She was just a child back then who found herself in a situation that required her to play the role of an adult. She played the part well, but I must admit I toned down her immaturity when I wrote the first book of this series. I don't say that to sound mean. In no way was she a bratty or bad teenager, but she was definitely still a teenager.

As all birthmothers do, she sacrificed her own instinctive will when she handed that beautiful little baby to us. We watched her heart break in two, leaving half of it here in Idaho while taking the other half back to Mississippi. We naturally felt guilty about that. We wished we could take that away. We ached along with her.

Teenagers tend to mature quickly, so every time she came to visit it was like we were dealing with a new Brianna. For an adoptive couple like us, one of the greatest gifts she could possibly give us would be to allow us to watch her mature and progress in life.

Brianna flew out to see us once a year for the first handful of years. Sometimes she would come alone. Other times she came accompanied by a family member who was excited to meet us in person. I was especially fond of the visit when Ira was three and Brianna brought along her own father. He had been extremely opposed to the idea of adoption when he first learned she was pregnant, but he has been solid over the years. It was a joy to have him in our home for those days.

Through the gift of hindsight, I look back on how wonderful another particular visit had been that seemed like a disaster at the time. Ira had come down with a high fever just as Brianna arrived to town. We had planned all kinds of activities and adventures for those four days, but all of those ideas were squashed by the need to stay home with our sick boy. The reason this turned out to be a blessing was because we could see how much that snuggle time meant to Brianna.

Ira has always been highly active. He was never one to just nestle up next to someone like Hazel would do. Especially when he was younger, he was not much of a snuggler. So this was the first time since he was an infant that she could just wrap her arms around him without him becoming restless after sixty seconds. Since we had become so secure in our relationship with Brianna, it was a delight to simply watch them cuddle up together and stay that way through an entire movie. I guess we learned during that trip that some of the greatest joys in life are found by slowing down and merely appreciating each other's company.

That fifteen-year-old who wrote us that cute letter almost ten years ago has matured into a remarkable woman. She graduated from high school with stellar grades and went on to study nursing. We have always found it funny that the birth-mothers of both of our children chose the same career path. Brianna has been married for a couple of years now and has since left Mississippi. They now live in Virginia.

Brianna and Jammie have become even closer as years have gone by. While adoption was the thing that brought us together in the beginning, they regularly talk over the telephone just like sisters, and oftentimes adoption never even comes up in their conversation. She has always been a beautiful part of our family. We are excited to see what the future has in store for Brianna and her husband, and we love that we get to be part of her family as their story unfolds.

5

A LIFELONG CALLING

As Jammie and I were going through the adoption process, we saw the need for more adoption advocacy in the world. We felt strongly that God was calling us to be out there to help educate people on how difficult the adoption process hurdles are. I do believe that it is a good thing there are so many hurdles in order for parents to adopt. If that were not the case, our nation would have a lot more trouble with child trafficking. But why does adoption have to be so extremely expensive?

Along with helping to bring awareness about the difficulties of the process, we have felt like God has called us to be a voice for the beauty and challenges of open adoption. Most people I run into do not have a realistic grasp of what open adoption is like. How could they? It is such an unusual lifestyle that those who have not been closely connected to it could not possibly understand. We did not understand before we got involved either.

That feeling of being called to speak led me to write out the story of our first adoption experience. To be completely honest, I did not have plans to do anything with that manuscript when I wrote it. Within a month of finishing the first draft, I was at an author's convention with a different manuscript in hand hoping to find an agent or publisher interested in my new fiction novel (I write fiction under the pen name N. G. Simsion). I was able to catch the attention of one publishing company's CEO while she was taking a coffee break between classes. It did not take very long before she rejected my novel, but we continued with small talk after my pitch. As it turned out, she had a soft spot in her heart for adoption because of her close connection to it. I mentioned to her that I had written out our experiences after adopting our son and she told me I should bring it to her on the second day of the conference.

To say that manuscript was still a rough draft would have been an understatement. I spent all evening and late into the night getting it a little bit closer to being presentable, but by the time I handed it over to her it was still a mess. To make a long story short, the CEO read the manuscript and was about to reject the book outright, but the lady in charge of marketing talked her into giving it a shot. This put Jammie and me on a whole new pathway because I now had a team of people coaching me on how to reach a maximum number of people through activism. Releasing my book was only a part of the way we reached the community.

I got to know a lot of wonderful people as I sat on discussion panels and taught adoption education courses. Although

Jammie is not a birthmother, she worked with caseworkers to help organize and facilitate birthparent support groups.

The day our relationship with Darcie went into a tailspin by posting too much information on our web page was the day we began to pull back on our public advocacy. We had been living and breathing adoption nonstop for three years straight. Because discussions on our web page could quickly and often get heated, we had to keep a perpetual eye on how the discussion of the day was going in order to make sure our page maintained a welcoming atmosphere—all day, every day. Once or twice a month we were preparing for teaching a class or helping to organize a big adoption event with a local charity.

We were doing all of these things on top of navigating our own complex adoption relationships and figuring out how to be good parents. We had known when we began that we could not do it forever. When we had started, we did not know how long we would ride that exhausting advocacy train, but we knew we had to keep a close eye on whether or not it ever overpowered the aspects of adoption that were most important to us: our children and their birthparents. When Darcie left that scathing letter on our doorstep, we knew we had pushed that envelope too far and it was time to pull back.

We felt good about the timing of this decision from the amount of attention our web page required. Since we had put so much time and tears into that page, we were not about to let it fade into nothing—not after all the good it had been able to accomplish over the last few years. We prayed fervently about what to do with it, and we both knew there was only one person we trusted to take over. She has done an amazing job at serving the adoption community by keeping that page going over the years.

Over the next year and a half, we continued to be part of the adoption advocacy world by participating on panel discussions and teaching a class here and there. When our adoption agency made some needed changes to their programs, we decided that would be our time to pull back even further.

Although it had been a mistake we made with Darcie that first changed our adoption advocacy path, our main focus regarding advocacy had always been to monitor how it would affect our children. The larger our audience grew, the more we knew our advocacy could push them into a spotlight they may or may not embrace. That would have been the last thing we wanted.

On top of that, our plan has always been to ensure our children feel like they are in charge of their own adoption story. During their first few years, we made all of the decisions based primarily on what we felt best. As Ira and Hazel grew a bit older and they began to react and interact more, we have had to reanalyze our focus. Now, we always ask for their input when we are making decisions regarding their adoption relationships. Our goal has always been to prepare them for the day when those reins are handed over to them so they can make all of those decisions on their own.

Ira and Hazel process their situation very differently. Hazel thinks about her birthparents often and brings them up in conversation regularly. Ira is not like that. He enjoys the little things, like when Jammie hands him her cell phone to send Brianna a happy birthday text message or a quick video chat on Birthmother's Day (the day before Mother's Day), but he does not spend nearly as much time thinking about these things as his sister does. In fact, it was not until just about two months ago that Ira walked into our room late in the evening and asked, "What is my birthdad like? Have you met him?"

Ira has a picture of his birthmother on his dresser next to his bed, and Hazel has pictures of her birthmother and birthfather's whole family, but we do not have a good picture of Daren for his dresser. Ira has never had a text message conversation with Daren or visited with him on a video chat.

For thirty minutes, Jammie sat cross-legged with him right there in the middle of the floor and had a beautiful heart-to-heart about anything he wanted to discuss regarding adoption. We had always tried hard to make sure he knew the door was open for that discussion, but, unlike his sister, this was the first time he ever instigated it on his own. I sat on the edge of the bed and offered my feelings here and there, but I mostly just smiled at the sight of them sharing this moment. She talked to him about how he has two younger half-sisters now through Daren's side. She talked about some of the good things Daren has done and sugarcoated some of the reasons why we have not been in contact much with him over the years.

As unfortunate as our relationship with Daren has been over the last few years, this moment with Ira made me glad that door has remained open a crack. Someday Ira will be old enough that he can decide for himself what he wants to do with that relationship, but that will be another hurdle for another day.

6

THIS IS WHO WE ARE

A fifteen-year-old girl we knew from church came to us one day and told us she was pregnant. She hung her head low as she said, "I was raped. I want you two to raise my baby."

We stood there with mouths agape as she talked about all of the terrible things going on in her life—how she was being abused at home where she lived with her grandma and uncle, the way the boys were verbally attacking her all day at school now that she began talking publicly about her rape, and her need to get out of the situation she was in. What a mess!

We took her straight to one of our church leaders to help sort out the situation. By the end of our discussion, we decided on a plan to get her out of there. Jammie and I agreed to allow her to stay in our home for a week as we sorted through some long-term options.

We knew from the start that we were not going to adopt this girl's baby. As soon as she began pouring out her soul, we knew that the adoption relationship that would be built upon this foundation was going to be incredibly delicate and even more complex than those we already had. We felt our role in this story would be to remain close to her through it all and we learned firsthand how important it is for us to have a bit of personal space for the adoption relationship to remain healthy. That would be too difficult to navigate while living a block away from all of this girl's family. On the other hand, our time as adoption advocates meant we knew of many wonderful couples right off the top of our head who would be over-the-moon excited to adopt this child and were strong enough to handle such a complicated situation.

I remember like it was yesterday the moment we all stood in the living room of that young girl's grandmother to have an intervention. Telling this grandma that her home was unfit for raising a teenager was one of the most uncomfortable things I have had to be part of. I knew this woman—not well, mind you, but we attended the same church. I did not know whether to be angry with her at the life this teenager was enduring or to feel sorry for her when I saw the hurt in her eyes.

We left that house with enough clothing for a week and drove straight to our house.

We tried our very best to give her the best emotional support possible. Jammie encouraged her to attend the same birthmother support group Brianna had attended when she was expecting Ira. Within a few days, however, it became apparent that Jammie and I needed to have a private discussion about our situation.

"How long ago did she say the rape took place?" I asked as Jammie and I walked together hand-in-hand around our neighborhood.

"Two months ago, I think she said," Jammie said.

"That's what I thought."

"Why?"

"Because something is off. I can't say for sure or to what extent, but not everything she is saying can possibly be true. She told me today that the doctor said she was having twins—a boy and a girl. And she said he told her that at her appointment a few weeks ago."

Jammie sighed. "Yeah. That's not possible to know this early in a pregnancy."

"Do you think she is really pregnant?" I asked.

"I have been wondering that myself. It's not exactly the kind of thing you call someone out on unless you're absolutely sure."

"Right." I pondered what to say next, since even voicing these next words on my mind made me feel guilty for thinking them. "At this point, I'm not even sure the rape ever happened."

"Again, it's not exactly the kind of thing we can just call her out on without being sure. The last thing a rape victim needs are more people saying they don't believe her."

By the end of the week, we did end up confronting her about it. We had to. Her story was changing so much that we knew it could not possibly be true. As much as we felt like she played us for fools, the worst part of it all was that she had been dragging the name of one her schoolmates through the mud with this false rape accusation.

She admitted the rape never happened. She admitted she had never been pregnant. The abuse and neglect she said had been happening at home was also made up. When it came down to it, she was just another case of a teenager wanting to get out of the house and live with someone else. Most teenage girls have wished for that at some point in their life, but this one took it to the extreme. She knew we had especially soft hearts for birthmothers and thus could see a way to take advantage of us.

This was the only time someone tried to manipulate us, but it was not the only time our hearts were sent into a frenzy. It was not the only time someone came to us for help with an unplanned pregnancy. Over the next five years, although we had already decided we were finished adopting now that we had two children, we were asked three more times to adopt someone's child. Two of those times we knew it would be best to refer them to one of the other hopeful adoptive couples we knew. The third time we actually agreed to adopt the child, but none of those three adoptions ever took place.

Some people are so shocked by the reality of an unplanned pregnancy that they decide early on in their pregnancy that they need to place their child for adoption. But as those nine months progress, it becomes very common for the mother-to-be to decide to raise the child herself. Adoption has continually become more and more rare.

Especially as political debates have heated up over the years regarding late-term abortions of babies who are mature enough to survive outside the womb, I am saddened by the fact that adoption is so rare. I do not think for a second that all women with unplanned pregnancies should place that child for adoption. I do not think it is right to even suggest that all single women need to consider it, but I sincerely wish adoption was more commonly a part of people's everyday conversation.

The truth is that, for every adoption that takes place, there are ten pregnancies ended by means of abortion. Being a man who sees everything in this world through my adoption lenses, I am saddened by that statistic.

There was a scene in *Open Adoption, Open Arms* in which Jammie and I attended a mandatory adoption preparation class. As we were socializing with some of the other hopeful adoptive parents, I quickly recognized a couple who had been in some of those classes when we adopted our first time around. I made some form of comment to them, assuming incorrectly that they were back to adopt again like we were. By the sad look in their eyes, I knew I had made a mistake even before they informed me they were still waiting to adopt for the first time.

We felt incredibly guilty about that. Many of the couples with whom we attended classes had been waiting since before we adopted the first time and here we were back to do it again.

Years later, I remember very well one afternoon when I was sitting quietly at a desk in the back corner of the public library working on one of my fiction novels. I noticed the familiar face of another woman I had known from the adoption world.

I took my hands off the keyboard and greeted her. "It's so good to see you again," I said. "I have lost touch with a lot of the awesome couples we used to see in our adoption classes since we don't teach them anymore. How are things going?"

She turned her eyes away for a moment before saying, "We took our name off the waiting list. We tried for nine years, but never got selected."

"I'm so sorry," I said. This fate was not new to me. I knew that was the reality for many of the couples we had worked with through our years of advocacy.

"We couldn't see the point in spending a thousand dollars to have our homestudy done every time we needed to renew. But more than that, we just gave up, I guess. A person can only hold onto that hope for so long and feel defeated every time we see someone else adopt."

I wish I could say I had some awesome words of comfort for her that day, but that would be a lie. I felt terrible for her, especially since their profile had been on the list when Jammie and I began the process and were there long after we had successfully adopted twice. I do not think the average person realizes how many couples give up after years of trying. Over that final year when Jammie and I were working closely with one of our local adoption agencies, there were eighty couples in the state of Idaho hoping to adopt through that agency. Only twelve adoptions took place that year.

We do not spend time monitoring a discussion board on a web page like we used to, but we feel like our calling to be adoption advocates is a lifelong pursuit. That call to act will manifest itself in a variety of ways as we pilot our family, but we will never keep our mouths closed.

There have been many times in our life when we have wished we could just be normal, but "normal" is not in the cards for us. There is a reason we have pictures of our children's birth families displayed in our home. They are family and we love them, and not only when times are easy.

Our family tree is unique. This is not only what we do. This is who we are.

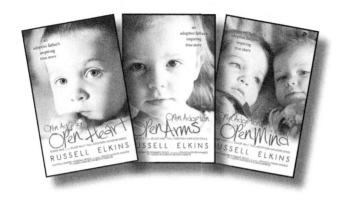

the **GLASS HALF-FULL ADOPTION MEMOIRS** *series:*

Open Adoption, Open Heart
the story of Rusell and Jammie's first adoption

Open Adoption, Open Arms
the story of Russell and Jammie's second adoption

Open Adoption, Open Mind
an interesting addition to Russell and Jammie's story
six years down the road

About the Author

Russell was born on Andrews Air Force Base near Washington, D.C. Along with his five siblings, he and his military family moved around a lot, living in eight different houses by the time he left for college at age 17. Although his family moved away from Fallon, Nevada, just a few months after he moved out, he still considers that little oasis in the desert to be his childhood hometown.

Russell moved to Idaho after graduating from Brigham Young University in Provo, Utah. He is captain of his men's league softball team, die-hard fan of the Oakland Athletics, avid disc golfer, fiction writer under the name N.G. Simsion, and guitar player/singer with a band he formed with his brother called *The Two in the Middle*.

Above all, Russell loves God and his family.

Printed in Great Britain
by Amazon

25116169R00033